THE
ARTHRITIS
EXERCISE
BOOK

Gentle, Joint-by-Joint Exercises to Keep You Flexible and Independent

Gwen Ellert, R.N., B.S.N.

Gillian Parker, P.T., Consultant   Foreword by Barry Koehler, M.D.

CB
CONTEMPORARY
BOOKS
CHICAGO

Library of Congress Cataloging-in-Publication Data

Ellert, Gwen, 1952–
    The arthritis exercise book : gentle, joint-by-joint exercises to
keep you flexible and independent / Gwen Ellert ; foreword by
Barry Koehler.
       p.   cm.
    Rev. ed. of: Arthritis and exercise. c1985.
    Includes bibliographical references.
    ISBN 0-8092-4094-7 (pbk.)
    1. Arthritis—Exercise therapy.   I. Ellert, Gwen, 1952–
Arthritis and exercise.   II. Title.
RC933.E46   1990
616.7′220624—dc20   90-37142
                                                CIP

Note:
Before embarking on any program or activity in this
book, be sure to consult your physician. The author
and publisher assume no liability in connection with
this program.

Illustrations by Dave Hancock

Published by Contemporary Books, Inc.
Two Prudential Plaza, Chicago, Illinois 60601-6790
Manufactured in the United States of America
International Standard Book Number: 0-8092-4094-7

This book is dedicated
to my parents,
Lew and Bernice Ellert.

CONTENTS

FOREWORD

The various forms of arthritis constitute the commonest reason for chronic disability. While prevention or cure for the more than one hundred different rheumatic diseases continues to elude us, virtually everyone with arthritis can expect improvement with a well-designed treatment program. Arthritis treatment usually involves one or more of several modalities, including physician care, education, medication, exercise, joint protection, and surgery. This book focuses on exercise, an area in which the individual with arthritis is particularly called upon to become his or her own therapist.

The importance of strong muscles to give support to diseased joints cannot be overemphasized, for both daily functioning and pain relief. As the author rightly observes, the information in this volume should complement, not substitute for, assessment and advice of a physiotherapist. Exercising has all the excitement and appeal of brushing your teeth, but, like this important aspect of dental health, the arthritic patient's exercise program should be an integral part of each day's activities.

I believe this book will provide an additional stimulus for the individual with arthritis to incorporate, into his or her daily activities, an exercise regimen.

Barry E. Koehler, M.D., F.R.C.P.(C), F.A.C.P.
Former Medical Director
The Arthritis Society, B.C. and Yukon Division, Canada

ACKNOWLEDGMENTS

For Medical Review: At the Arthritis Society, B.C. Division—Dr. B. E. Koehler, Medical Director; Bonnie Denford, M.Ed., Director of Physiotherapy. The Educational Team: Catherine Busby, B.Sc. (O.T.), Occupational Therapist; Bruce Clarke, R.P.T., Physiotherapist; Kathryn Duke, R.N., B.A.; as well as Pamela Pethick, R.N., B.S.N.; Dr. H. B. Stein, Rheumatologist; Dr. R. W. McGraw, Orthopedic Surgeon; Dr. S. Hemming, Medical Health Officer, and Dr. F. Hemming, Aviation Medicine.

For Technical Review: Christine Allan, Editor; Anna Daniels, B.Ed; Lorraine Ewonus, B.Ed.; Gerald and Susan Pinton, Marketing and Public Relations Consultants; Michael Parker, Vice President, Vertigo Computer Imagery; George Ewonus, Master of Education; William Preston, Executive Director, Arthritis Society, B.C. Division.

For Support: Thank you also to the many people who gave their input and support for the project and to my family and friends for their encouragement throughout this project and for their supporting me through the acute stages of arthritis.

A special thank you for the time and talent donated by the production team: Ilka Abbott, whose experience as a librarian was invaluable; Dave Hancock, who drew these special characters for the book as well as spending additional hours working on the technical format; Michael Kluckner, author and artist, whose publishing experience made my life much easier; and Carole Vince, who patiently typed and retyped without even a sigh.

I also would like to thank my treatment team: Dr. Howard B. Stein, Rheumatologist; Gillian Parker, Physiotherapist; Jackie Henwood, Occupational Therapist; and Dr. Robert W. McGraw, Orthopedic Surgeon.

Check with your doctor before beginning this or any exercise program.

INTRODUCTION

I wrote this book for people with arthritis, both young and old, and for the inactive who would like to *improve with caution* the flexibility and strength of their bodies. While the main focus is on rheumatoid arthritis, the exercises are generally applicable for anyone with any form of arthritis. The book is designed to prevent the damage that can be caused by improper daily exercise, the wrong exercise, or too much of any one exercise, and it reinforces the importance of an exercise routine.

In this age of the beautiful body, exercise looks so easy. Just put on your matching shorts, top, and jogging shoes and head off to exercise class. But it is not as easy as it may look. When I first began trying to exercise, I had trouble opening my eyes in the morning and getting out of bed on time! I tried setting the alarm clock half an hour early, but even the promise of feeling better afterwards was not enough motivation to make me get up.

I decided to try exercising at the end of my day

when time was my own. But I was so glad to have made it through the day that I did not want to feel as if I had to do anything else!

For some reason I believed exercise must be easier for people without physical disability or pain to contend with. Not true! They may progress faster to optimum fitness, but they still have to have the willpower to get up that half an hour earlier and not to give in to the desire to collapse when they have finished their day's routine, be it at home or at work.

It is true, people with arthritis may be more fatigued. You may have the morning pain or stiffness. But it still is the willpower that counts: the willpower to do something *for yourself*, to take that initial step to becoming as fit as you can—however boring, however painful.

There is nothing I can do to give you the willpower to exercise. This book is for those who recognize the need for exercise, would like to exercise, but presently cannot keep up with the fast pace of exercise groups. We need a much more controlled and individualized method of stretching and strengthening our bodies.

There is no easy way to start to exercise. It will help, however, to know why you should exercise, and to realize that a person with arthritis has more to gain from it than someone already able to move easily and free of restrictions.

Exercise should be approached on a day-to-day basis. You should have a good understanding of what your minimum ability is and how you can build to your maximum ability. As you build up to your maximum, a knowledge of the composition of a joint and the way it works with various muscles to produce motion will help you understand what each exercise is doing for you, and why.

1
GETTING STARTED

If you think that exercising sounds like a surprising idea for a person with arthritis, you are not alone. In fact, until relatively recently even doctors recommended immobilizing or resting a sore joint. Today, however, though rest is still important in the overall treatment of the disease, research has shown the enormous benefits of following an exercise program such as this, which is specially designed to keep undue pressure off joints. This program will help those with both rheumatoid arthritis and osteoarthritis, which are two of the most common of the more than one hundred types of the disease.

Rheumatoid arthritis, for an as yet unknown reason, causes the body to send antibodies to a joint, producing the painful swelling associated with the disease. Instead of healing the tissue, the white blood cells attack and begin to destroy joint tissues, cartilage, and eventually the bone. Osteoarthritis, commonly associated with old age or sports injuries, also involves breakdown of cartilage and other joint tissue, and although it does not cause the inflammation of rheumatoid arthritis, the disease is painful and limits one's movement.

Keeping movement in a sore joint to a minimum is a natural reaction; the result, however, is that the muscles surrounding the joint "atrophy" or waste away. Consequently the muscle can no longer support and help the joint move as it should. Weak muscles must work overtime, causing even more pain.

Exercise, first of all, will increase circulation, which helps in diminishing the painful swelling around the joint. Although joint cartilage is eroded and destroyed during the course of the disease, research is finding that exercise encourages the body to help repair this damage. Perhaps most importantly, exercise helps to build up atrophied muscles surrounding a joint. Strong muscles are able to take excess weight off sore joints, provide support, and help the joint move. Lastly, and more generally, exercise promises more energy, a sense of well being, and even weight control.

THE DISEASE PROCESS

The following diagram shows the anatomy of a normal joint:

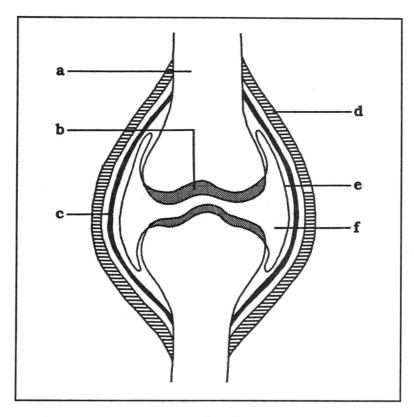

a = bone

b = articular cartilage

c = joint capsule

d = ligaments

e = synovial membrane

f = joint space containing synovial fluid

Bone gives shape to and supports the body. It offers protection to some organs (e.g., heart and lungs) and gives a point of attachment for the muscles.

Articular (joint) cartilage covers the surface or ends of the bone at the joint, providing a smooth surface for ease of motion.

The joint capsule encloses the whole joint and, with the **ligaments** which reinforce and strengthen it, provides support to the joint.

Synovial fluid is a somewhat thick fluid which is produced by the synovial membrane and contains water and nutrients which lubricate and nourish the joints. The lubrication is necessary to reduce friction between the cartilage surface and the bone ends.

The synovial membrane is a thin layer of tissue which lies under the joint capsule and lines the synovial cavity. This membrane produces synovial fluid.

The joint space is enclosed by the bones and the joint capsule and contains the synovial fluid.

The diagram on page 3 shows a normal joint. You may already know that the word *arthritis* simply means "joint inflammation." It is important to understand the difference between normal joint inflammation and inflammation caused by rheumatoid arthritis.

NORMAL INFLAMMATORY RESPONSE

Inflammation is the way the body reacts to anything that has invaded or injured the tissue. Normally when disease or injury affects a joint, inflammation also occurs in that joint.

The body directs special fluids to the affected area. These fluids contain cells and chemicals which help to destroy whatever caused the injury and to repair the damaged tissue.

With all this activity going on, the affected area becomes swollen and hot. (Hot because of the increased blood supply to the area; swollen because of the extra fluid in the affected area).

This normal inflammatory reaction uses up body energy. Therefore, you may find you are more tired than usual while the body is trying to repair itself. During this time, it is a good idea to rest the injured area.

RHEUMATIC INFLAMMATORY RESPONSE

With rheumatoid arthritis, the cause of the inflammatory reaction is not known. As with normal inflammation, the body responds by sending special fluids to the area. However, in the process of trying to heal the tissue, the synovial membrane begins to swell and thicken. It produces cells and chemicals which start to destroy the membrane, the cartilage, and, eventually, the bone.

As the inflammation causes more swelling, the joint capsule and ligaments supporting the joint are stretched.

At this stage of the disease, your joint is hot, swollen, *painful.* You do not want to move this sore joint. Therefore, after a short period of time, you will find the muscles around the affected joint become weaker. Now, instead of just one problem—arthritis—you have two problems, the second being muscle atrophy.

This process does not necessarily create a downhill cycle. The disease tends to flare (become active) and then go into remission (become inactive). During a flare-up, it is important to exercise properly and move your joint through the entire range of motion.

Motion helps to maintain the movement you have.

Then, when the disease is in remission, you can increase your range and strength.

Ideally, you should exercise *every joint every day*, to some degree, especially when the disease is active. Although it is essential to move all affected joints daily, motion must be determined by the degree of heat, pain, and swelling at a particular time. Excessive and improper motion may aggravate an inflamed joint.

Also, when the joint is hot and swollen, the joint capsule is stretched. Over time this stretching could cause the surrounding tissue, capsule, and ligaments to lose their ability to support the joint. Therefore, once you have exercised the joint, you should support it by using specific aids or "supports." These supports may help to ease the joint stress so that you are not stretching or straining the ligaments while they are vulnerable.

Finally, because medical science cannot eradicate the cause of the disease and cure it, the available treatments only help control the disease. It may take time to find the best treatment for you. Be patient. Work with your doctor and other members of the treatment team—such as the physiotherapist, nurse, occupational therapist, or dietitian—to find the treatment that is right for you.

The important thing is to get this treatment in the early stages of your disease—*before permanent damage has occurred.* In most cases the effects of the disease can be lessened by anti-inflammatory medication, rest, and exercise as recommended by your treatment team.

EXERCISING TO FIGHT THE DISEASE

This book will cover two sets of exercises.

The first set is stretching, designed to maintain and improve your *range of motion and flexibility.*

Daily range of motion is essential for all ages and in all stages of your disease. These exercises will help to maintain the range that you already have. As the disease starts to come under control, they will help to increase your range.

The second set of exercises is strengthening, designed to maintain and improve your *muscle strength*. As your strength increases, you will find that your energy level will also increase. Because the muscles will take some of the stress of moving off your joints, soon you will find that you are moving more easily.

Reasons for Exercise

- Proper exercise for each joint will help to maintain or increase the range of motion, or *flexibility*, so you will be able to move more freely.
- Strong muscles will take some of the pressure off joints that are damaged or painful, allowing you to move more efficiently and more comfortably.
- Exercise will indirectly have a beneficial effect on your weight. If your disease is very active, you may have lost weight. Once the disease is under control, the weight may come back. This is good, but with a less active lifestyle, you may find that over a long period of time you will end up carrying more weight around than you need—and that is hard on your joints.
- Exercise will improve your self image. You will be doing something for yourself which will eventually make you feel stronger and more agile—opening up your world again.

THE APPROACH

Before exercising a joint, you must know how far the disease process has progressed. Check each joint and *classify* it as category 1, 2, 3, 4, or 5, according to the chart on page 13.

Decide which exercises you will do. Be realistic. You should not attempt to do everything all at once. *Always exercise the worst joints first.* A good way to start is to set aside fifteen minutes twice a day. Some people find that doing the stretching exercises in the morning and the strengthening exercises in the evening works well.

If the disease is very active and you are not used to exercising, you may only be able to exercise your three worst joints in fifteen minutes. As you improve, you will be able to do more. If for any reason you miss a few days in a row, start back at a lower level.

Remember you are starting on a project for yourself that may take some months to become a part of your lifestyle. You are the one who will benefit from the discipline needed to do your daily exercise. You may miss a day or two, but do not let that cause you to give up your program.

Approach the exercises one day at a time. Remember every little bit helps. Do the exercises regularly. *Do not substitute* an activity for an exercise. Most daily activities do not use your full range of motion.

Listen to your body. Your guide to knowing whether or not you have exercised too much is pain. Two hours after having done your exercises, joint pain should be the same as or less than it was when you started. Increased pain means that you did too much. The next day *decrease* the number of repetitions.

When exercising, the following guidelines are important:

- Be sure you do the movement as it is written: for example, with legs bent, or toes pointed.
- Exercise with control. Do not rush through your exercises, but rather move slowly and properly, concentrating on the muscles being used.
- Remember to breathe correctly—oxygen is important to the body and in particular to the function of the muscle. When you exercise, you should breathe out during the exertion phase of the exercise. For example, if lying on your side and doing a side leg raise, exhale as you lift your leg (exertion phase) and inhale as you relax your leg and bring it to the floor (relaxation phase). Your breathing should be from the diaphragm—your abdomen should move as you breathe, not your shoulders.

Finally, check your posture throughout the day! Good posture while you are sitting or standing means keeping your head up, your shoulders back, your seat muscles pulled in and firm. Good posture is an easy way to help the well-being and function of your entire body, and you should feel good as you maintain it.

Remember, check with your doctor before starting this or any other exercise program.

PREPARING FOR EXERCISE

You may find that you can increase your range of motion by first decreasing the pain as much as possible. Therefore, after you have assessed your joints, try one or all of the following:

- Twenty minutes before you start to exercise, take your pain medication.
- Ten minutes before you start to exercise, apply an ice pack (or bag of frozen peas) to your hot and swollen joints.
- Put on some music with a definite beat and rhythm to keep the pace going and take your mind off the discomfort.

READING THE SKELETON DIAGRAMS

Throughout the book you will see diagrams of an odd-looking skeleton with circles showing where the joints are (except for the spine).

The *black circles* on these diagrams indicate the joints that the exercises will stretch (primary joints). The *gray circles* indicate any joints that may also move (secondary joints). You should be aware of, and cautious in, the movement of all the involved joints.

You may have difficulty exercising the primary joint if a secondary joint is inflamed. Try to find a comfortable position for the secondary joint. Start the exercise. If the joint is too painful, then do the minimum number of repetitions and move on to the next exercise.

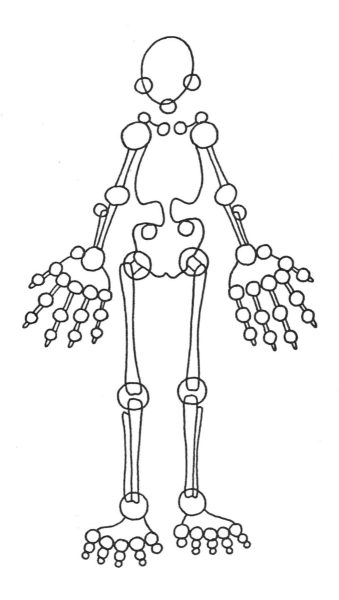

2
STRETCHING

Covered in this section are the neck, shoulders, elbows, wrists, hands, hips, knees, ankles, toes, and back. Assess each joint and classify it as category 1, 2, 3, 4, or 5. Then repeat the following stretching exercises as indicated below. That is, if your elbow is a category 3, a joint that is a little swollen but not hot and not painful, repeat each elbow exercise five times.

Category	Ellert-Parker Joint Classification System	Repeat Exercise
1	Normal healthy joint, never been affected	10 times
2	A joint at one time affected by arthritis, but which today is cool and neither swollen nor painful	10 times
3	A joint that is a little swollen, neither hot nor painful*	5 times
4	A joint that is swollen and hot or painful*	3 times
5	A joint which has been replaced (at present, this category does not apply to the neck, wrist, or back)	5 times

*When doing your stretching exercises at these levels, push your joint just past the point of discomfort.

SITTING AND STRETCHING

The following exercises should be done while sitting in a straight-backed chair with a firm seat and no arms (i.e., a kitchen chair that does not swivel). Sit with your buttocks against the back of the chair.

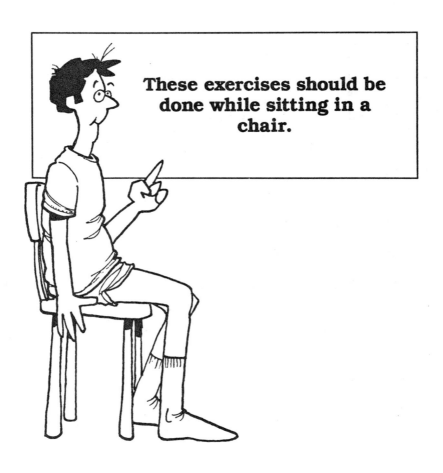

These exercises should be done while sitting in a chair.

NECK EXERCISES

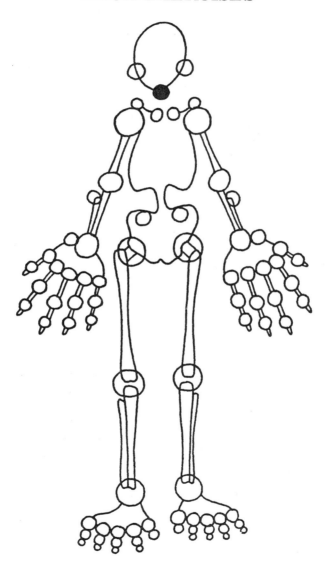

Some Activities Involving the Neck

- Almost any activity, even ones as simple as having a conversation with a few friends, or watching television
- Driving, reading, and sewing

Lifestyle Tips

- When you are required to hold your head in one position for a long time, for example, when you are reading, watching TV, riding in a car, bus, or airplane, remember to:
  1. Be aware of positioning. Hold your head in the neutral position, not bent forward, as forward bending will cause undue stress on the neck and may result in pain across the back of the head.
  2. Stop what you are doing and go through the neck movements every half hour.
- Position of your neck at night is important. When lying on your side, use one soft pillow that can be tucked well into your neck for support.
- Collars for neck problems are available, but *do not* buy one without advice from your doctor. It is very important that you have the right type of collar for your specific problem.
- Recurring headaches across the back of the head may be a warning of joint inflammation in the neck. If your neck is persistently painful, let your doctor know.

Exercise Hints

- When doing these exercises, do not force your head down to the shoulder, or your chin over your shoulder.
- Just relax and slowly move your neck.
- When you are lying down and doing the neck exercises (page 53), your muscles will be more relaxed and you may be able to get a little extra range of motion.

Neck Bend

Look straight ahead. Bend your left ear to your left shoulder. Then bend your right ear to your right shoulder and lift your head back up to the center.

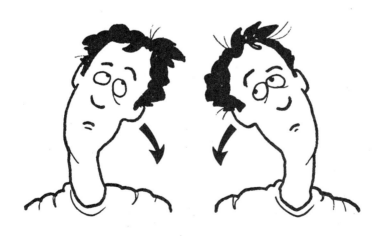

Neck Turn

Turn your head left so that you are looking over your left shoulder, then turn it right to look over your right shoulder, then turn back to the center.

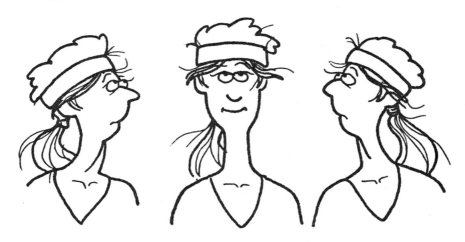

Caution

Avoid putting your neck in either the flexed (chin to chest) or extended (tilting head back) position.

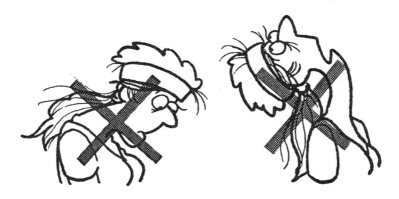

Neck/Spine Stretch

Sit up straight, pull your shoulders back, tuck your chin in, and imagine someone is pulling on a string attached to the top of your head.

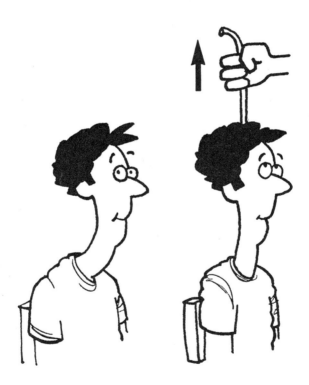

SHOULDER EXERCISES

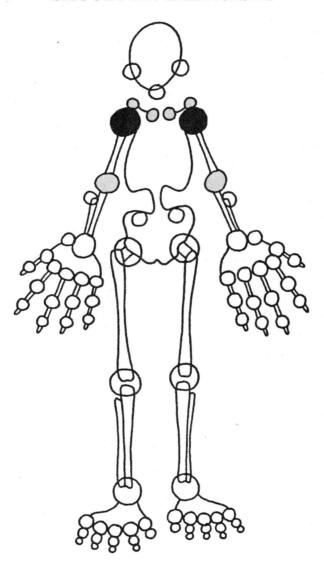

Some Activities Involving the Shoulder

- Combing hair; putting on a coat
- Reaching for things (on a desk, in a cupboard)
- Holding a steering wheel when you are driving
- Tucking in your shirt

Exercise Hints

- The mid-range, when your elbow is straight and your hand is at shoulder level, causes the greatest stress on the shoulder joint. Therefore, if your shoulder is painful, you may wish to put your hands together and/or bend your elbow while doing the exercises. It will decrease the stress and make the exercises a little easier to do.
- If your elbow is sore, first put your elbow in a comfortable position and then exercise your shoulder.
- If your shoulder is painful, you may find that the lying down shoulder exercises, on pages 54–57, are easier for you.

Lifestyle Tips

- When you put on a coat, shirt, or sweater, put your sore arm in the sleeve first.
- Adjust your cupboards and shelves so that frequently used items are on the lower shelves.
- If you lie on your side at night, you may find it comfortable to tuck a small pillow up near the shoulder under the arm on which you are not lying.

Shoulder Lift

Sit with head facing forward. Lift your left shoulder up while keeping your left arm by your side. Then drop your left shoulder down, lift your right shoulder up, and drop it down.

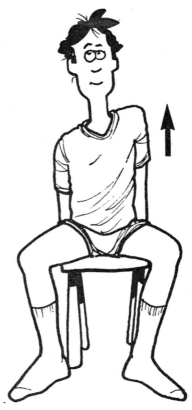

Frontward Arm Lift

Start with both arms straight down by your sides. Keep your palms toward your sides with thumbs up. Lift your arms forward and up to your ears. Then slowly lower them back to your sides.

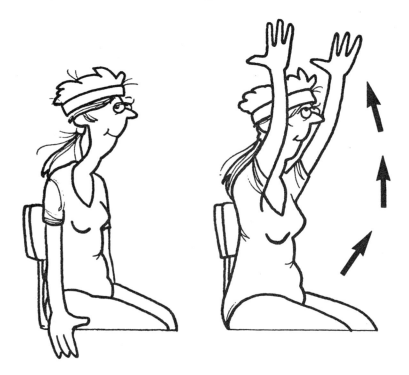

Hands Behind

Put your hands behind your head and pull your elbows back. Then return your arms to your sides. Now put your hands behind your back and slide your thumbs up as high as you can.

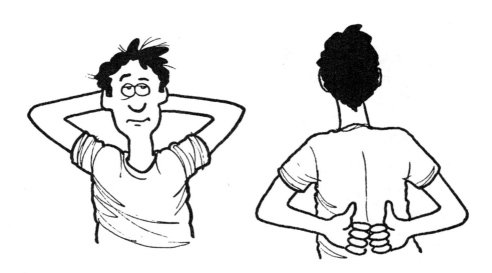

Outward Arm Lift

Start with both arms straight down at your sides, palms facing down. Lift your arms out to the sides (as high as your shoulders). Then turn your palms up and lift your arms up above your head.

Now slowly return your arms to the height of your shoulders. Turn your palms down and bring your arms back to your sides.

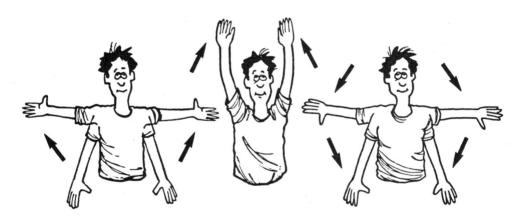

ELBOW EXERCISES

Do each exercise first with your left elbow and then with your right elbow.

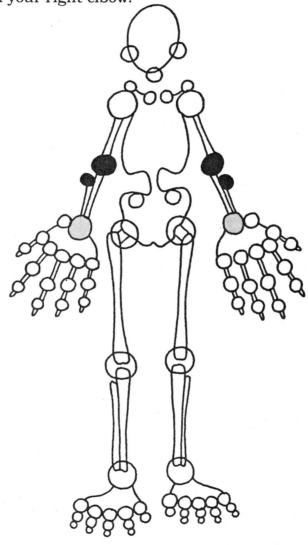

Some Activities Involving the Elbow Joint

- Lifting heavy or bulky items
- Personal hygiene and grooming (shaving, brushing teeth)
- Eating
- Drawing, painting, gardening
- Answering the telephone
- Opening doors
- Using the gear shift in a car

Exercise Hints

- Support your forearm with your other hand.
- Adjust your arm to get your elbow into a comfortable range.

Lifestyle Tips

- If you drive, try to avoid using a gear shift car.
- If you must transport heavy things like groceries or suitcases, use a buggy or cart with wheels.
- If you must lift a small child, have the child at your waist level (i.e., on a table or a couch) when you are standing. Then lift.

Elbow Bend

Start with your arm straight down at your side. Bend your elbow, bringing your hand up so your fingers can touch your shoulder. Then slowly lower your arm back to your side.

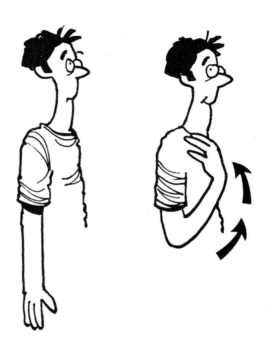

Elbow Roll

Start with your elbow bent at 90 degrees and tucked into your side. Point your thumb toward the ceiling. Now roll your thumb to the outside (palm face up) as far as you can. Then roll your palm down so that it faces the floor. Finally, roll your palm back to the starting position.

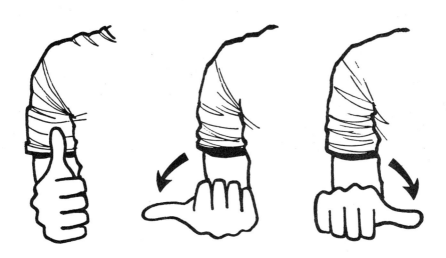

WRIST EXERCISES

Do each exercise first with your left wrist and then with your right wrist.

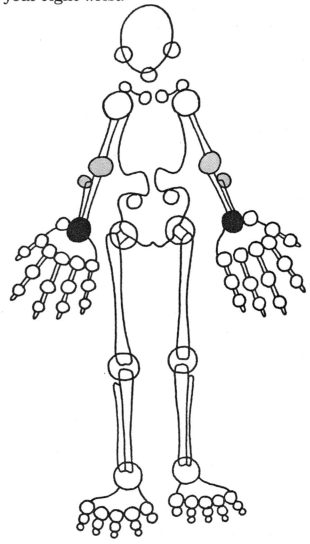

Some Activities Involving the Wrists

- Personal hygiene
- Cooking and eating
- Receiving change
- Writing or typing
- Opening a door with a key

Exercise Hints

- Keep your fingers relaxed when doing these exercises.
- Holding your forearm still with the other hand may help you to get your wrist to its maximum range.

Lifestyle Tips

- Never wring out a wet cloth. Instead, wrap the cloth around the tap and then twist the cloth with both hands.
- Use two hands for lifting pots and pans.
- Split the loads you have to carry into smaller bundles (e.g., carry one cup of coffee with two hands instead of one tray with four cups on it).
- For very painful wrists, custom-made splints may help relieve stress and pain and therefore help prevent permanent damage. Contact your doctor or therapist for more information.

Wrist Bend

Have your elbow bent and tucked into your side, with your palm toward the floor. Bend from the wrist and point your fingers down to the floor. Then bend from the wrist and point your fingers up to the ceiling, pulling back as far as you can.

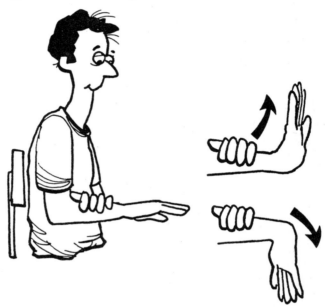

Wrist Circle

Keep your elbow tucked into your side and your hand out in front of you, fingers straight. Do not move your forearm (hold forearm still with other hand). With your hand, draw the largest circles you can in the air, first going one way then the other—remember only your wrist should be moving.

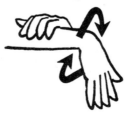

HAND EXERCISES

Do each exercise first with your left hand and then with your right hand.

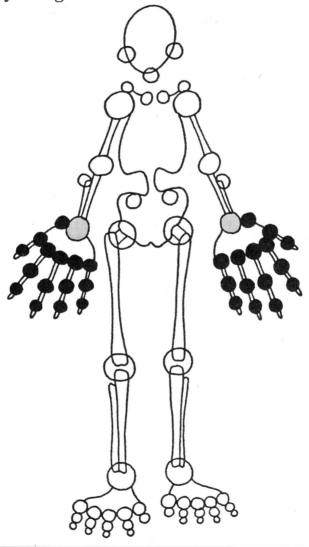

Some Activities Involving the Hands

Many of the same activities that involve the elbows and wrists involve the hands.

- Grooming and eating (holding utensils)
- Doing up buttons/zippers
- Opening doors
- Writing or typing
- Handling money

Lifestyle Tips

- Do not rest your chin on your hand, or push up on your knuckles to get up from a chair. These actions encourage the drifting (shifting away from the thumb) of your fingers.
- Pad or extend the handles of your utensils, pots, taps, keys, tools, car steering wheel, etc., so you will not need to grip the handles as tightly.
- A button hook may help you do up your buttons.
- Pin a long ribbon to the end of a zipper to help open or close it.
- Choose a fatter pencil or pen when writing.
- Carry small, light loads—even if you must make more trips.
- Use two hands to pick up and carry heavy items.
- When shaking hands with a person, take his or her hand first and grip only the fingers.

Exercise Hints

- Move and stretch each finger properly. Remember there are 15 joints in each hand.
- Fingers affected by the disease may tend to drift away from the thumb. It is important to be aware of exercising your hands properly to prevent this drifting.
- Strong grip exercises, such as squeezing a ball, should be avoided.

Finger Curl

Gently tuck the tips of your fingers into their inside base. Keep your knuckles straight, making sure that they do not move. Then stretch them back out.

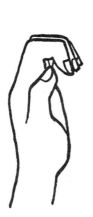 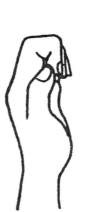 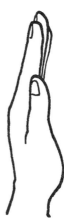

Loose Fist

Start with your fingers extended, then gently tuck them into the palm of your hand. Close your hand to make a loose fist. Then slowly stretch your fingers back out straight.

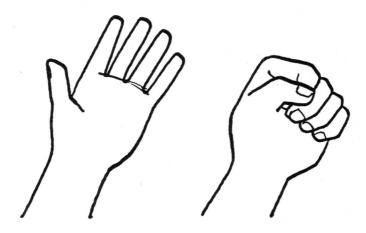

Finger Touch

Touch your thumb to the tip of each finger of your hand.

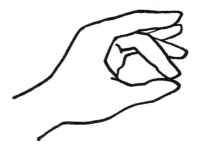

Thumb Stretch

Stretch your thumb as far away from your fingers as possible and then relax.

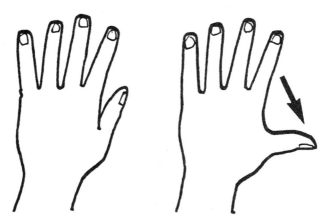

Finger Slide

Start with your hand flat on a surface, thumb and fingers together and straight. Slide thumb away from fingers. Then slide index finger toward thumb, long finger to index (keeping the rest of your hand still). Slide your ring finger to the long finger and baby finger over to ring finger. Then relax.

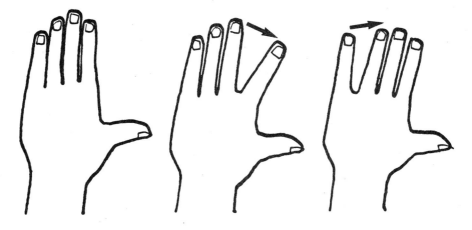

HIP EXERCISES

Do the exercise first with your left leg and then with
your right leg.

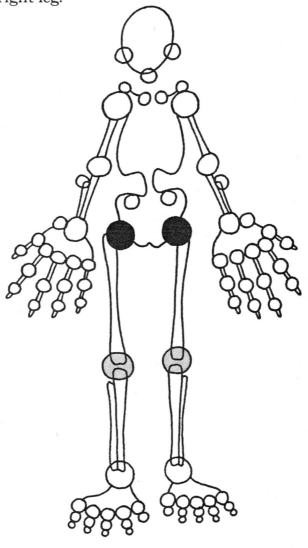

Some Activities Involving the Hips

- Getting in and out of a bathtub or a car
- Putting on your socks and shoes
- Walking and climbing stairs
- Sitting and bending

Exercise Hints

- If you have a hip replacement, you may wish to obtain the *Total Hip Replacement Owner's Manual* (see page 104).
- For maximum benefit, totally relax your leg muscles between each leg lift.
- Do not do these exercises too quickly. Be sure to stretch a little farther than you think you can.

Lifestyle Tips

- A stick with a hook on the end of it will help you to avoid bending over to pick things up.
- Sit on firm, high seats.
- At night you may find it helps to sleep with a pillow between your legs when lying on your side.
- Avoid climbing stairs if your hips are sore.
- Do not cross your knees if your hips are sore, as this puts unnecessary stress on the hips.
- If you need to push yourself up off a chair, push from your palms, not your fingers. Be aware that you do not want to stress your fingers and cause them to drift.
- Avoid sitting for long periods. Walk or shift your position every half hour.

Hip Bend

Start with your hands resting on your lap and your back straight. Lift your knee to your chest as far as possible. Then slowly lower your leg and put your foot back on the ground.

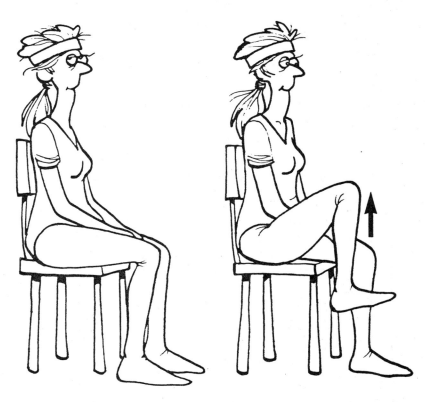

KNEE EXERCISE

Do the exercise first with the left leg and then with the right leg.

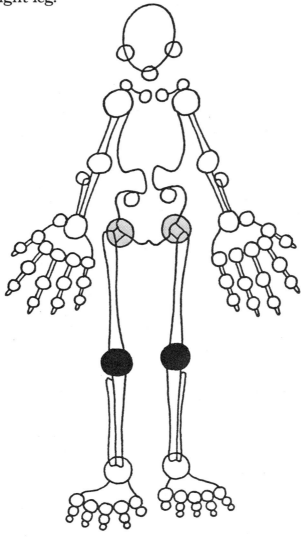

Some Activities Involving the Knee Joints
- Getting up from a chair and sitting down
- Walking
- Climbing stairs

Exercise Hints

- If you have a knee replacement, you may wish to obtain the *Total Knee Replacement Owner's Manual* (see page 104).
- It is very easy to lose some range in your knee without even noticing it. You can cope very well with some degree of loss, but if the knee does not straighten fully, the stress on the knee increases. It is very important to concentrate on straightening your leg as much as possible.

Lifestyle Tips

- Sit on firm, high seats.
- Avoid stairs when your knees are sore.
- Walking is good exercise for your heart and lungs, but do not overdo it or push yourself. End the walk *before* you get tired so that you can do the walk the next day as well.
- Build up the seats that you sit on by:
  1. using a solid cushion on a firm chair
  2. using a cushion when in your car
  3. raising the height of the seat of your toilet
- When on your feet a lot, wear low-heeled shoes with good support.
- Avoid standing still in any one spot for any length of time.
- Sit on a high stool while you wash dishes, prepare food, or work at a workbench.

Knee Stretch

Lift your foot up as high as your knee, keeping your toes pointed at the ceiling and your leg as straight as you can. Hold this position and try to straighten a little more. Now bend your knee and pull your foot back as far as possible under your chair.

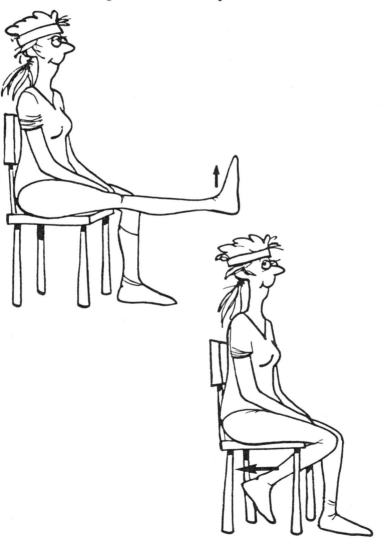

ANKLE EXERCISES

Do each exercise first with the left ankle and then with the right ankle.

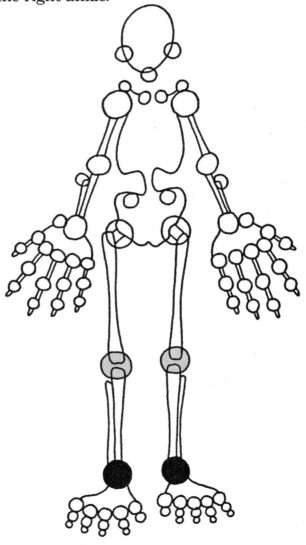

Some Activities Involving the Ankle Joint

- Walking, especially on uneven ground
- Driving a car
- Standing
- Climbing stairs

Exercise Hint

- This is another joint in which you may not notice a loss of range. Therefore, concentrate when you are exercising in order to reach that maximum stretch. You will feel it across the front of your ankle when you point your toes and up the back of your leg when you pull your foot up.

Lifestyle Tips

- Avoid sitting still in any one spot for any length of time.
- Sit on a high stool while you wash dishes, prepare food, or work at your workbench.
- Keep your feet up whenever possible.
- Wear good shoes with low heels, good arch supports, and laces or velcro fasteners. Insoles may be helpful as well. Save your party shoes for a party where you can sit down.
- If you must go to a meeting or reception, find a chair so you do not stand for a long period.
- When you go for a walk, be sure you walk on even ground, not on rocks, sand, or ground with potholes.

Ankle Bend and Stretch

With your leg in a position most comfortable for you
(relaxed, or extended, or anywhere in between), point
your toes down as far as possible (feel the pull on
your ankle). Then pull up and point your toes toward
your head.

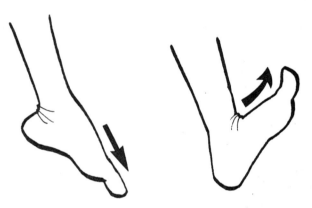

Ankle Circle

Draw a circle in the air with your big toe. Be sure to keep your leg still and move only your ankle. Repeat, circling in the opposite direction.

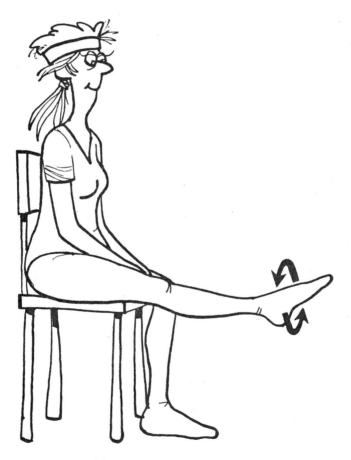

TOE EXERCISE

Do the exercise first with the left foot and then with the right foot.

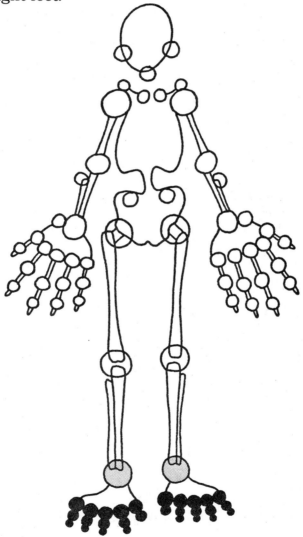

Some Activities Involving the Toe Joints
- Climbing stairs
- Balancing when you walk
- Prolonged standing

Exercise Hint

- You can see from the diagram on the previous page that there are a number of joints in your foot. Be sure to exercise every one of them. A problem with any one joint can cause you to protect that foot. If you do not take proper care of that joint, eventually you may have trouble with the whole foot.

Lifestyle Tips

- As with the ankles, your shoes are extremely important to your toes. Badly fitting shoes or insoles may do more harm than good. If you need to have a pair of custom-made shoes or insoles, contact your nearest arthritis center for a recommendation of someone who can make shoes or insoles for arthritic feet.
- With any pair of shoes, be sure that you have adequate room for your toes.
- Properly fitted running shoes can be an alternative to conventional oxfords or heavier shoes as many running shoes provide good internal and external support.

Toe Stretch

Start with your feet flat on the floor. Keep your toes straight and on the floor as you lift your arch and slide the toes back toward the heel. (This is a very subtle movement—your foot actually moves very little.) Relax. Then stretch your toes apart as far as possible.

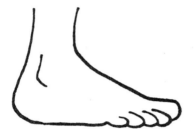

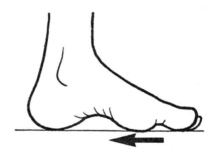

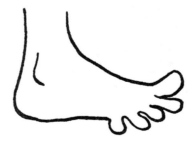

BACK EXERCISES

This is the section of the book where you would expect to find the back stretching exercises. These have not been forgotten, but on purpose have not been included, since the back is a very special area.

There are some very basic trunk exercises on pages 86 to 91. But if you do have a back problem, then you will need advice from your doctor or therapist as to which exercises you should do for your particular problem.

LYING DOWN AND STRETCHING

The following exercises should be done while lying on a bed or, if possible, lying on the floor.

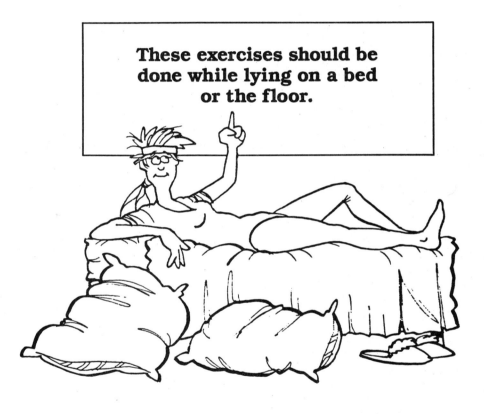

These exercises should be done while lying on a bed or the floor.

NECK EXERCISES

Refer to pages 15–17 for secondary joints that will move and exercise hints.

Neck Turn

With your head as flat on the bed as possible, turn your head first to the left, then back to the center. Now turn to the right and back to the center.

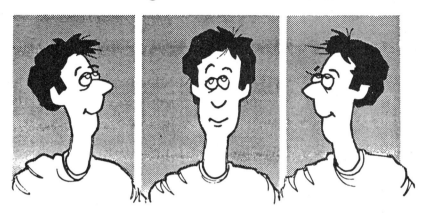

Neck Bend

Slide your left ear toward your left shoulder, then slide your head back to the center. Now slide your right ear toward your right shoulder, then slide your head back to the center.

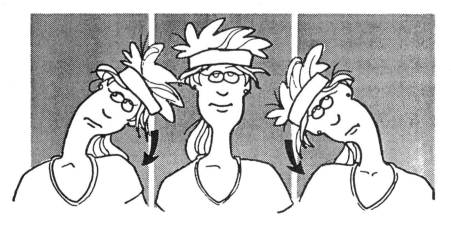

SHOULDER EXERCISES

Do each exercise first with your left shoulder/arm and then with your right shoulder/arm. Refer to pages 20 and 21 for secondary joints that will move and exercise hints.

Arm Slide

Start with your arms at your sides. Slide one arm out from the side and up to shoulder level. Keep your arm straight, turn your palm toward the ceiling, and slide your arm up to touch your ear. Now slowly slide your arm back to your side.

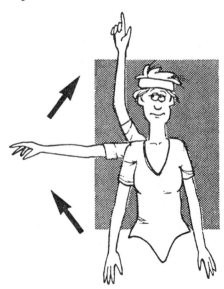

Arm Lift

Scoot down into the middle of the bed. Start with your arms at your sides. Now lead with your thumb and slowly raise your straight arm up above your head, then lower your arm behind your head to touch the bed. Then reverse the motion and slowly return your arm to your side.

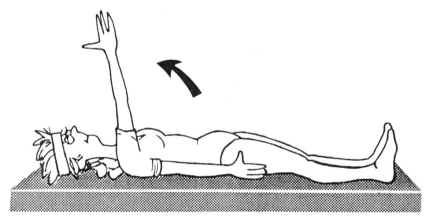

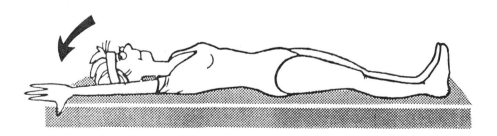

Elbow Turn

Bend your elbow 90 degrees, tucking it into your side. Slowly move your forearm as far away from your body as possible. Then bring it back forward and move the same forearm across your stomach and back to your side.

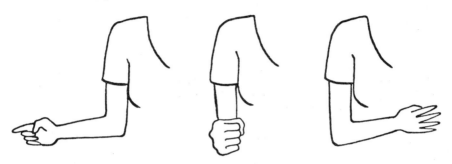

Shoulder Lift

Lift your shoulder up as far as possible to your ear (do not bend your head down to your shoulder). Slowly lower your shoulder, feeling the pull down as you lower it.

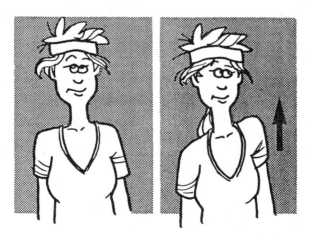

Elbow Stretch

DO THIS EXERCISE WITH CAUTION. Do not put any pressure on the back of your neck. Put your hand behind your neck and lift your elbow up as high as your shoulder. Then, keeping your elbow at shoulder level, move your elbow behind your head and shoulder, pressing your elbow into the bed as far as possible. Feel the stretch and then slowly relax.

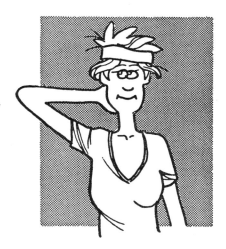

HIP EXERCISES

Lie on your back and do each exercise first with your left leg and then with your right. Refer to pages 38 and 39 for joints that will move and exercise hints.

Leg Slide

Start with both legs together and straight. Lead with your heel and keep toes pointed up to the ceiling. Slowly slide your leg out to the side, then bring it back to the center. (Make sure that you are sliding your leg—do not lift your leg off the bed).

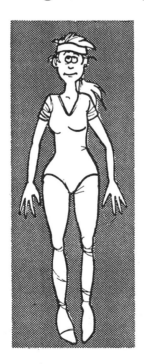 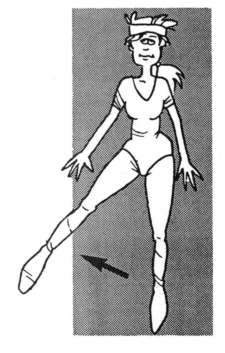

Foot Roll

Bend one knee—keep the other straight. Using the leg that is straight, bend that ankle and point that foot to the ceiling. Slowly roll that foot out.

Then bring your foot back up and point your toes to the ceiling. Now roll the foot in, then bring it back to point to the ceiling.

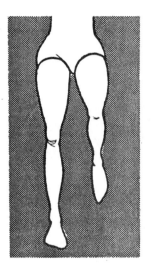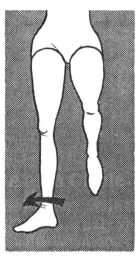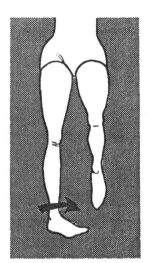

Bent Leg Lift

Bend both knees. Lift your left knee up as close to your left shoulder as possible. Now slowly lower your leg back so that your foot is back on the bed and your knee is still bent. Repeat with your right knee.

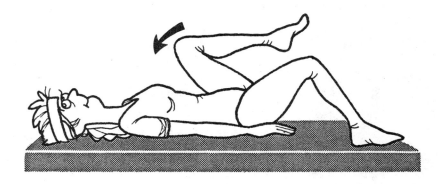

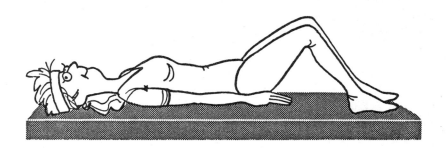

KNEE EXERCISES

Do each exercise first with your left leg and then with your right leg. Refer to pages 41 and 42 for joints that will move and exercise hints.

Heel Slide

With the backs of your knees touching the bed, bend one knee, keeping your heel on the bed. Bring the heel as close to your buttocks as possible. Then slowly slide your heel back out so that your leg is straight.

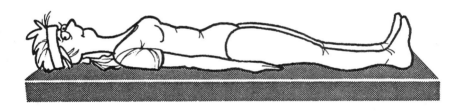

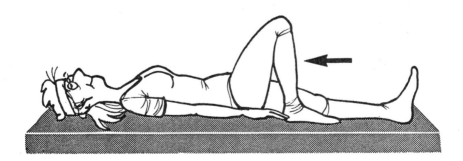

Straight Knee Stretch

With your leg straight, push the back of your knee into the bed. At the same time try to lift your heel up off the bed and point the big toe at your head.

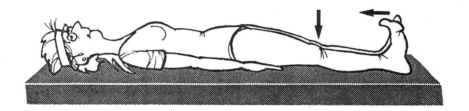

3
STRENGTHENING

The key to strengthening the muscle surrounding an arthritic joint is repetitive movement, against gravity, with a "concentrated hold" to make that muscle work. When you do stretching exercises, you rhythmically move through the range of motion, then back to your starting position. Now, with the strengthening exercises, you want to move your body part into the correct position, tighten the muscle, and hold it tightly by concentrating on it for ten seconds. After ten seconds, you should completely relax the muscle and put your body part back into the starting position. You should do a "concentrated hold" on each muscle group at least three times. Put your body in a position that will be comfortable for you and do the best you can when you tighten that muscle.

UPPER BODY

Strengthening your upper body involves working with your shoulders and arms—shoulder, elbow, and wrist joints.

Refer to the joint category 1, 2, 3, 4, or 5 which you selected for each joint, and repeat the following upper body strengthening exercises as indicated below. For example, if your shoulder is category 4, a joint that is swollen and hot or painful, repeat each shoulder exercise three times.

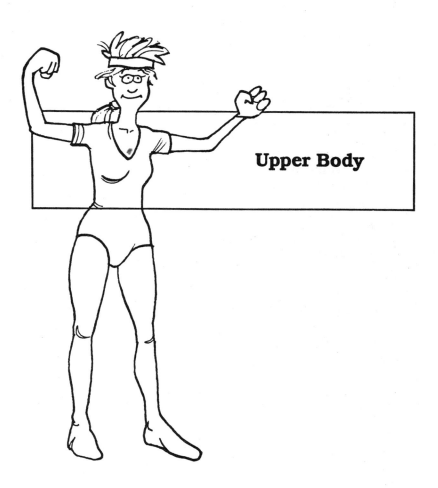

Upper Body

Category	Ellert-Parker Joint Classification System	Repeat Exercise
1	Normal healthy joint, never been affected	10 times
2	A joint at one time affected by arthritis, but which today is cool and neither swollen nor painful	10 times
3	A joint that is a little swollen, neither hot nor painful	5 times
4	A joint that is swollen and hot or painful	3 times
5	A joint which has been replaced (at present, this category does not apply to the neck, wrist, or back)	5 times

SHOULDER MUSCLES

Do each exercise first with your left shoulder and then with your right shoulder.

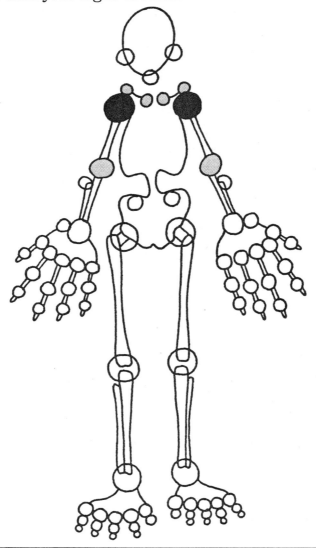

Exercise Hints

- You may wish to place a small towel between your shoulder and the wall to add a little padding.
- Concentrate and feel the muscles around your shoulder as they tighten. If you are doing the exercise properly, you should be using only your shoulder and upper arm muscles.

Lifestyle Tips

- Extend the handles on your personal hygiene items (e.g., hairbrush, comb, toothbrush, etc.)
- Most drug stores carry a back brush, which will help you with washing your back.
- Buy clothes that open in the front instead of ones that button up the back or pull over your head.
- Use extended drinking straws.
- Use a dressing stick (a stick with a hook on the end) to help pull on your clothes or coat.
- A well-placed safety pin attached to a long ribbon will also help you pull on your clothes.
- A "reacher"—a stick with a curve like a cane— will help you reach for things.

Forward Shoulder Press

Stand in a doorway and set one foot slightly ahead of the other to steady yourself. Stand so that the front of one shoulder and arm is set against the door jamb. Keep that arm straight by your side, push forward against the door jamb, and hold the tightened muscle for six to ten seconds. Feel your upper arm and shoulders tighten, then relax.

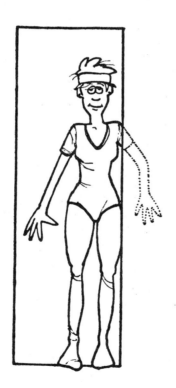

Side Shoulder Press

Stand with one shoulder next to a wall and your foot three inches from the wall. You may keep your arm straight or bent at the elbow. Without moving your body, try to push the wall away by using your upper arm. Push and hold that muscle tight for six to ten seconds.

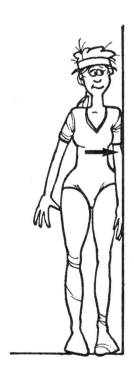

Backward Shoulder Press

Stand with your back against the wall and your heels three inches out from the wall. You may keep your arm straight or bent at the elbow. Without moving your body, push the back of your upper arm against the wall. Push and hold that tightened muscle for six to ten seconds and relax.

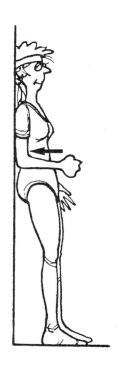

ARM MUSCLES

Do each exercise first with your left arm and then with your right arm.

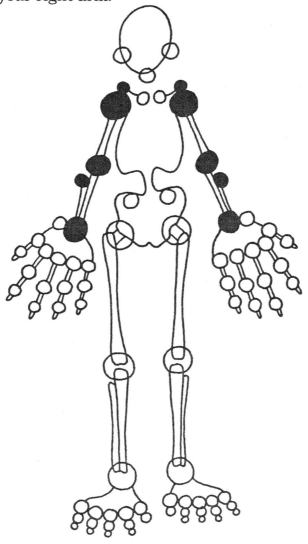

Exercise Hints

- Concentrate and feel the muscles contract. As you pull up on the table, the muscle on the front of your upper arm tightens. As you push down on the table, the muscle at the back of your arm tightens.
- If your shoulder or elbow is very sore, first find your most comfortable position or angle, then tighten the muscles.
- A small towel between the table and your arm will provide a little padding.

Lifestyle Tips

- If your hands are sore, you may find it helpful to put strap loop handles on things such as the oven door or drawers, etc. Then you can use your forearm to pull them open.
- A non-slip pad on your kitchen counter or workbench will reduce the stress required to stabilize an item.
- Loops of ribbon as handles on your bedclothes will help with adjusting your blankets.

Table Press Up

Sit down in front of a heavy table. Place the palms of your hands under the table (just above the wrists on your forearms) with your thumbs extended out against the table. Push up against the table with your palms. Hold the muscles tight for ten seconds, then relax.

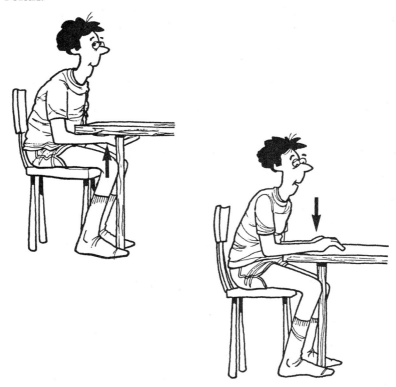

Table Press Down

Sit down in front of a heavy table. Place the palms of your hands on top of the table, with your thumbs stretching toward the ceiling, and rest your forearms (just below the wrists) on the table. Push down on the table with your palms. Push and hold the muscles tight for ten seconds, then relax.

LOWER BODY

Strengthening your lower body involves working with your legs—hip, knee, and ankle joints.

Again refer to the joint category 1, 2, 3, 4, or 5 which you selected for each joint, and repeat the following lower body strengthening exercises. That is, if your hip is category 3, then repeat each hip exercise 20–30 times.

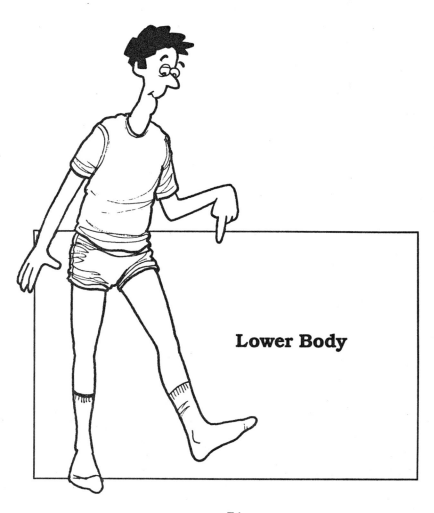

Lower Body

Category	Ellert-Parker Joint Classification System	Repeat Exercise
1	Normal healthy joint, never been affected	20–30 times
2	A joint at one time affected by arthritis, but which today is cool and neither swollen nor painful	20–30 times
3	A joint that is a little swollen, neither hot nor painful	20–30 times
4	A joint that is swollen and hot or painful	at least 3 times and no more than 10 times
5	A joint which has been replaced (at present this category does not apply to the neck, wrist, or back)	5 times

HIP MUSCLES

Do each exercise first with your left leg and then with your right leg.

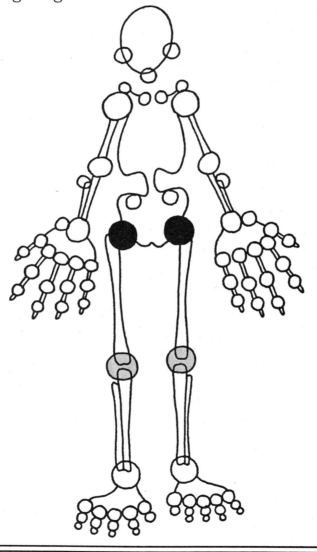

Exercise Hints

- With the Side Leg Lift, it is important to lift the leg about 10–12 inches off the bed, just high enough to make that leg muscle work without stressing your back. Tightening your stomach muscles will help support your back while your leg is in the air.
- With the Leg-Belt Press, the wider the belt, the more comfortable it will feel. A small towel between the belt and your leg may be helpful.
- The Back Leg Lift is designed both for stretching and strengthening the hip area. You may be more comfortable if you allow your feet to hang over the end of the bed and if you place a small pillow under your stomach to stop you from arching your back.
- If you have low back pain, you may wish to omit the Back Leg Lift.

Lifestyle Tips

- A long stick with double-sided tape on the end of it is helpful for picking small things off the floor.
- Long-handled reachers are available; check with a medical supply store.
- A cane may be helpful until the muscles are strong enough to provide adequate support for the hip joint. The cane must be the correct length and should be held in the hand opposite to the sore limb.

Side Leg Lift

Lying on your side, with the bottom leg bent, tighten the muscles above the knee (quadriceps) of the leg closest to the ceiling. Lift the top leg up in the air toward the ceiling. Hold for six to ten seconds, return to starting position, and relax.

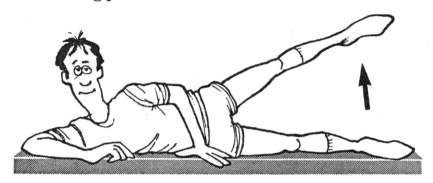

Back Leg Lift

Lie on your stomach, keep your leg straight, and tighten the muscle above your knee (quadriceps). Lift the leg into the air. Hold for six to ten seconds and relax.

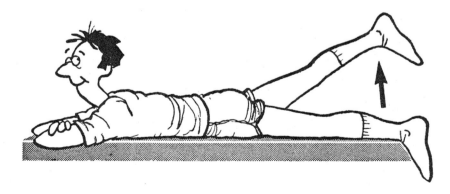

Leg-Belt Press

Using a belt, loosely strap your legs together above your knees. Lie flat. Keep one leg still and slide the other leg away from the still leg until the belt is taut. Hold six to ten seconds and relax.

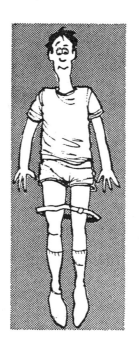 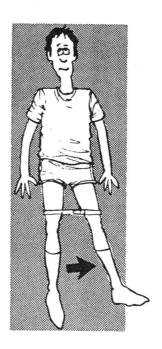

KNEE MUSCLES

Do each exercise first with your left leg and then with your right leg.

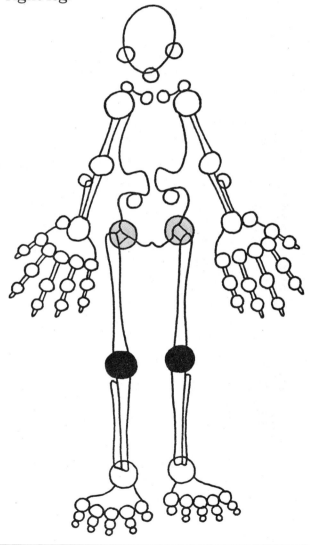

Exercise Hint

- With both of these exercises, if you set your hand on your thigh, you will be able to feel the quadriceps muscle tighten and work.

Lifestyle Tips

- You may find it helpful to raise the height of the toilet seat.
- A bathtub grab bar and tub mat will help you stabilize yourself as you move around in the tub.
- As with the hip, a cane may be helpful as long as it is the correct length and held in the opposite hand to the sore limb.

Knee Straighten

Sit in a straight-backed, firm-seated chair without arms. Straighten your leg and concentrate on tightening the muscle above your knee (quadriceps). Hold for six to ten seconds and relax.

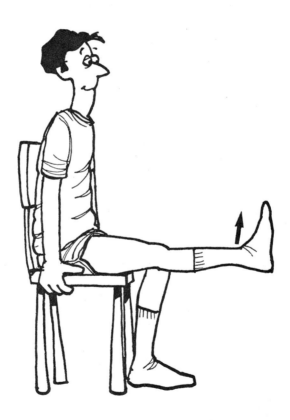

Heel Press

With your feet firmly on the ground and one of your legs directly in front of the chair leg, bend that leg back to the chair leg so that your heel touches the leg of the chair. Now push your heel against the chair leg for six to ten seconds and relax.

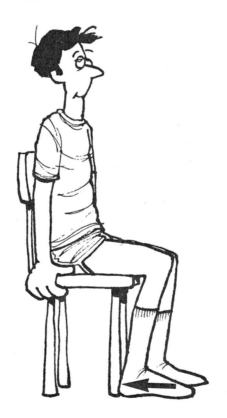

ANKLE MUSCLES

Do this exercise with both ankles at the same time.

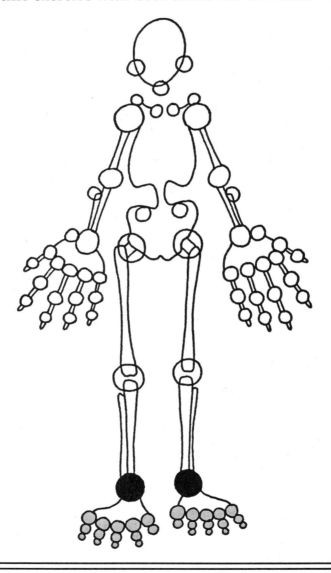

Exercise Hint

- Concentrate so that you are able to feel the muscle in the back of your lower leg (calf muscle) working.

Lifestyle Hints

- When your ankles are sore or swollen, put your feet up.
- Make sure that your knees are supported when your feet are propped up.
- Push pillows to the end of the bed, between the sheets, so that the top sheet and blankets do not put any unnecessary weight on your ankles.

Heel Lift

Hold on to something for support. Now go up on your toes so that you lift your heels about two inches off the floor, then slowly put your heels back onto the floor.

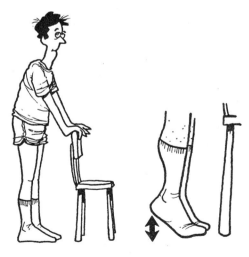

TRUNK

The trunk muscles include both stomach and back muscles. They provide support to your back and are essential for good posture. Strong stomach muscles will help you move from a lying to sitting position without pushing or pulling on painful upper limbs.

These exercises can also help improve your endurance. If you are able to repeat each exercise enough times to make you out of breath, your heart and lungs will get a workout as well.

Do these exercises as recommended, gradually increasing the number of repetitions. Remember, pain is your guide. If increased pain is still present two hours after exercising, decrease the number of times you repeat the exercise next time.

The trunk exercises require that you assess the comfort level of your back. The categories for assessing your back are:

1	pain-free
2	some discomfort
3	painful

1. Pain-free

If your back is pain-free, do all three trunk exercises. Start by doing each exercise 5 times, gradually increasing to a maximum of 30 times. If you remain pain-free, increase the number of repetitions by 5 times every three days. That is:

Day 1:   5 times each
Day 4:   10 times each
Day 7:   15 times each
Day 10: 20 times each
Day 13: 25 times each
Day 16: 30 times each (maximum)

2. Some discomfort

If your back feels a little painful or uncomfortable, you can do all three trunk exercises, but do not repeat them as many times. Start by doing each exercise 5 times, gradually increasing to a maximum of 15 times.

Day 1:   5 times each
Day 4:   10 times each
Day 7:   15 times each (maximum)

3. Painful

If your back is painful, the only exercise you should do is the Pelvic Tilt. Start by doing the exercise 5 times and gradually increase to 15 times. If you cannot do even 5 pelvic tilts, you should contact your doctor.

Pelvic Tilt only:

Day 1:   5 times
Day 4:   10 times
Day 7:   15 times (maximum)

Relax after each set of five.

Activities Involving the Trunk

- Everything you do involves the spine and trunk muscles. Therefore, be aware of the *posture* and *position* of your body at all times!

Exercise Hints

- Do all exercises smoothly and with good muscle control. It is better to do five properly than ten poorly.
- Do not push yourself if your back is painful.

Lifestyle Tips

- Posture! Posture! Posture! Good posture means sitting or standing with your head up and shoulders back, your seat muscles and stomach muscles pulled in and firm.
- When lifting anything, be sure to bend your knees and keep the object as close to you as possible. If your knees are painful, it may be easier to go down on one knee before lifting.
- When resting, lie with your knees slightly bent. A pillow under your knees may feel more comfortable. This position can help you relax your lower back.

Pelvic Tilt

Lie flat on your bed with knees slightly bent. Tighten your stomach muscles and push your lower back into the bed, tilting the pelvis backward as you tighten your buttocks. Hold for a count of five, then relax.

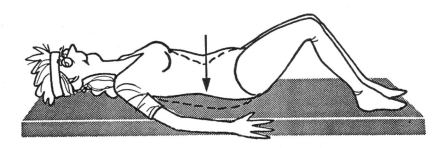

Head and Shoulder Lift

Lie on the bed or floor with knees bent and arms by your side. Now raise your head and shoulders about six inches off the bed and hold for a count of five, slowly lie back down and relax.

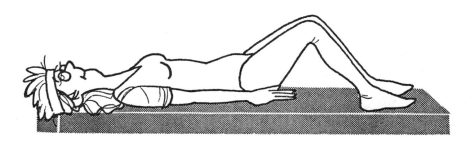

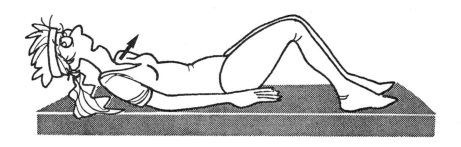

Knee-Pelvis Turn

Lie flat on the bed with knees bent. Keeping your knees together and both shoulders touching the bed, slowly lower both legs to the left to touch the bed, then bring them back to the center. Now slowly lower them to the right, touch the bed, and bring them back to the center.

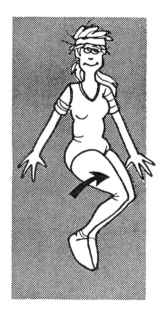 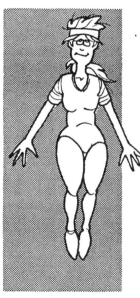 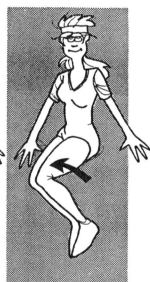

4
RELAXING EXERCISES

You have made it to the last group of exercises! Now relax and yawn—it is a terrific exercise for the jaw!

JAW RELAXATION

Lifestyle Tips

- Jaw pain may be described as an earache.
- If your jaw is sore, try to eat soft foods and cut your food into small pieces.

Jaw Stretch

Hold your head straight. Slowly open your mouth as wide as you can without forcing your jaw. Then slowly close your mouth.

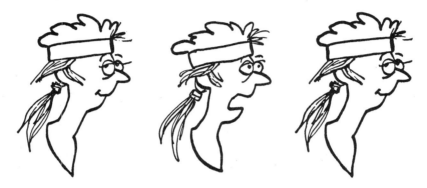

Exercise Tip

● You can check whether your range of motion is increasing or decreasing in this joint by using your fingers to measure how wide your mouth opens. Open your mouth as wide as you can and put your fingers in your mouth. Your fingers should be one on top of the other rather than side by side.

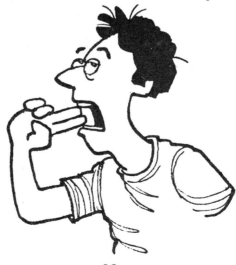

DEEP BREATHING RELAXATION
Rib Cage Breathing

Lie flat. Put your hands on your rib cage. Breathe in slowly for a count of three and feel your rib cage expand. Hold your breath for a moment. Then push all the air out of your lungs and feel the rib cage collapse. Then relax and repeat. Do this five times, then stop and rest for a minute. Now repeat another five times.

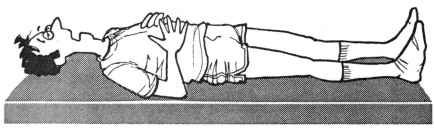

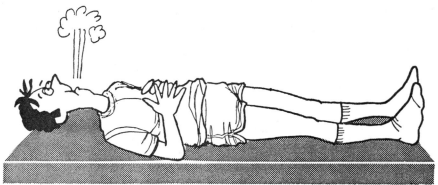

GENERAL RELAXATION
Whole-Body Tense and Relax

Lying flat, systematically tighten all your muscles. First curl your toes. Then tighten your knees, then your seat muscles. Next tense your shoulders. Now close your eyes tight.

Hold for a count of five, then relax your face, shoulders, seat, knees, and finally your toes.

If it feels good, you may wish to repeat this two or three times.

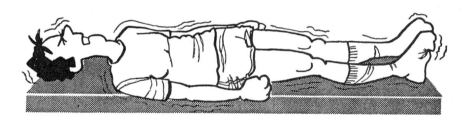

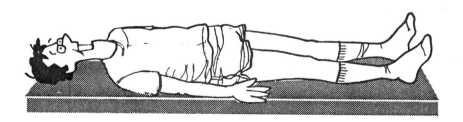

5
LEISURE AND TRAVEL

Some people are concerned about participating in various leisure activities or coping with travel when they have a disability. This section provides some information and suggestions on how you might approach these two important areas.

LEISURE ACTIVITIES

A person needs both a daily exercise program and leisure activities. The leisure activities encourage relaxation and social contacts. The daily exercise serves to maintain and increase your flexibility and strength. Hopefully, your daily exercise program will help you to increase your choice of leisure activities.

For some people, finding leisure activities that they can do and will enjoy may be a challenge. For example, if your favorite sports are tennis, water skiing,

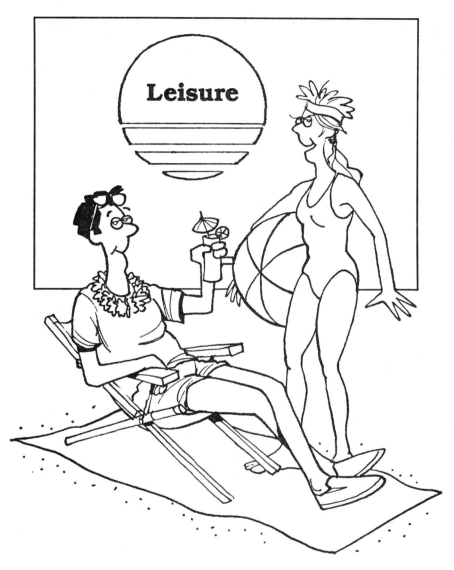

and snow skiing and you have some degree of joint damage in your legs or arms, there are better activities in which to participate actively. But if you enjoy a sport and do not want to give it up completely, then simply adjust the way you take part. You can "coach" from the sidelines, join in on the beach party, or meet with your friends after the ski lifts have shut down. Do not cut yourself out. You can continue to understand and enjoy the enthusiasm of others and their tales about the sport. It may not be your ideal way to participate, but it is better than no contact at all.

The only drawback with this type of participation in sports is that it does not provide the exercise that *you* need. So, while coaching from the sidelines, keep following your exercise program and, if necessary, look for new activities and hobbies.

Points to consider before participating in any leisure activities:

- Be honest with yourself. Consider if any of your joints are swollen or painful. Avoid activities or at least decrease activities which will cause extra stress or strain on the sore joints.
- Wear good shoes (i.e., golf shoes, walking shoes, running shoes, hiking boots). Proper support for your feet is essential and will help you to keep your body in proper alignment.
- Quick starts and stops, as well as constant twisting and turning, add a tremendous amount of stress to the lower body joints and back. Racquet sports are particularly likely to involve these stressful movements.
- You may be able to modify the way you do an activity in order to reduce the stress on the specific joints so that you can still enjoy the sport.
- Look over the lifestyle tips in the book and see if you can adapt them to your activity. Remember, if you behave yourself now, respect what your sore joints are telling you, and prevent unnecessary joint damage, maybe next year you will be in better shape to resume your normal activities!

Below is a list of activities ranging from singing to hiking. This list is meant to give you some new ideas about things you might try. Before you attempt any one of them, remember to consider the points I have just mentioned. Also, you may wish to decrease your involvement in something else for a while. That is, if you are already walking every day and want to start swimming as well, then decrease your walking. Try walking four days a week and swimming three days a week.

Art galleries	Ice/Roller skating
Billiards	Knitting/Crocheting
Bird watching	Macramé
CB radio/Ham radio	Musical instruments
Camping	Night school
Cards	Painting
Chess	Ping-Pong
Computers	Pottery
Cross-country skiing	Reading
Cycling	Racquet sports
Dancing	Singing
Fishing	Snow skiing
Flying	Stamp/Coin collecting
Gardening	Swimming
Gliding	Theatre
Golfing	Walking
Hiking	Weaving
Hot-air ballooning	Woodworking

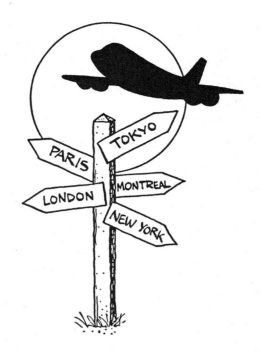

TRAVEL

When you travel, remember that although you know your own limitations, a stranger may not have even noticed them. If you need assistance, do not hesitate to ask for it! Most people in the tourist industry are very helpful. You are paying for a service, and they would like to make your journey as pleasant as possible. Also, other passengers are very obliging and will lift a bag off a shelf or help you with your coat—if you ask. If someone asked you for assistance, would you not help if you could?

There are many agencies that can provide travel information to people with special needs. Although the focus is generally directed toward people in wheelchairs, it is likely that these hotel chains, airlines, or tour companies will be receptive to accommodating others with special needs.

The following is a list of some sources of information when traveling with special needs:

- Travel Information Service
  Moss Rehabilitation Hospital
  12th Street and Tabor Road
  Philadelphia, Pennsylvania 19141-3099
  (215) 456-9603
    Provides information for handicapped travelers on accommodation, transportation, and tourist attractions in the U.S., Canada, and abroad.

- The Itinerary
  137 Bayonne Street
  Bayonne, New Jersey 07002
  (201) 858-3400
    A magazine dealing with various topics of interest to disabled travelers.

- The Hub, Physically Handicapped Service Center
  P.O. Box 4397
  St. John's, Newfoundland A1C 6C4

- *Access To The World: A Travel Guide
  For The Handicapped*
  by Louise Weiss
  Facts on File Publications
  New York, New York, 1983

- *The United States Welcomes Handicapped Visitors*
  Society for the Advancement of Travel for the
  Handicapped
  1012 14th Street NW
  Suite 803
  Washington, DC 20005

- Travel Agencies
    A few travel agencies specialize in travel for the handicapped. Ask the agent, before you make any arrangements, if the agency is familiar with ways of traveling for your special needs.

- Contact your local public health unit for information about shots that may be required or potential health problems in other countries (e.g., water or climate).

- Contact your local librarian to see if they have the above information or other sources of information.

POINTS TO CONSIDER WHEN TRAVELING

- If you are concerned about traveling and making your own arrangements, you may wish to travel with an organized tour group. The tour staff generally makes all your transportation and hotel arrangements, as well as ensures that your baggage is taken from one station to the next.
- When you book your ticket, be sure to let the agent know what your needs are (e.g., a seat near the washroom, a wheelchair, etc.)
- Be sure that you have enough travel insurance to cover any reasonable mishap that may occur (e.g., lost medication, hospitalization).
- Carry all medication with you. Do not put it in your suitcase in case your luggage goes astray. Ask your doctor for the following information about your medication, and then carry the information with you:

1. What is the generic (international) name for my medication?
2. What dosage do I take?
3. What are my normal blood levels?
4. Is there any other medical information I should carry with me?
5. Should I wear a medical alert bracelet?

- Take along your splints and aids, such as dressing sticks or tap turners. If you are staying in a hotel or motel, you can leave a note for the maid regarding certain items (e.g., ask that they do not turn the taps off too tightly and explain why).
- Use lightweight luggage with wheels. Take two small suitcases instead of one large one.
- Carry-on baggage should have a shoulder strap and, if possible, wheels. If your hands are sore, you will have another way to carry the bag.
- On long trips where they are sitting still for a long time (car, air, train, or bus), many people will tend to stiffen up, whether or not they have arthritis. Every half hour, exercise your ankles and toes and then, once every hour, do as many of the stretching exercises as possible. If you are traveling by car, stop every hour and walk around for about five minutes. As you walk you can do your exercises. Some exercises can be done in the car.
- Do not be too proud to ask an attendant for help if it would make things easier for you. You should save your energy for things that matter and times when no assistance is available.
- Ask for a wheelchair to transport you through the terminal. Attendants do not question why you want one—but do give them notice of your requirements. Again, save your energy for more important and enjoyable things.

ADDITIONAL READING

Most of these are pamphlets, but some are small books. The Arthritis Society puts out a number of publications besides those listed here, many of which are free. Those from the Arthritis Foundation are generally $0.10 per copy. Your family doctor may also have free pamphlets available.

The Arthritis Society
250 Bloor Street East Suite 401
Toronto, Ontario, Canada M4W 3P2

Aids and Adaptations $4.00*
Easy Is the Name of the Game $1.00
Basic Facts About Arthritis $0.70

The Arthritis Society: B.C. and Yukon Division
Vancouver, B.C., Canada V5Z 1L7

Lupus and You: A Guide for Patients $3.00
Your Hands—The Art of Self-Defence $1.50
Total Knee Replacement Owner's Manual $1.50
Total Hip Replacement Owner's Manual...... $1.50
MCP Joint Replacement—Owner's Copy $1.50
"My Mom Has Arthritis" Colouring Book..... $2.00
Straight Talk on Ankylosing Spondylitis $10.00

Note: Please add 15 percent for postage and handling. Payment must be enclosed with order.

*These amounts given are in Canadian dollars. U.S. residents should send either a money order in Canadian funds or a check that takes into account the current exchange rate.

The Arthritis Foundation
79 W. Monroe, Suite 510
Chicago, IL 60603

Systemic Lupus Erythematosus
Ankylosing Spondylitis
Psoriatic Arthritis
Polymyositis
Polymalgia Rheumatica
Bursitis, Tendinitis and Other Related Conditions
Unproven Remedies
Diet and Nutrition
Living and Loving

The following U.S. pamphlets are now also available from The Arthritis Society in Ontario at a cost of $0.20 each:

Facts About Gout
Facts About Inflammation
Facts About Osteoarthritis
Facts About Rheumatoid Arthritis

Prices are subject to change without notice.
Delivery—4 to 6 weeks.

ARTHRITIS ORGANIZATIONS

The Arthritis Society (in Canada) and The Arthritis Foundation (in the U.S.) are national, nonprofit, voluntary health organizations which depend on public support for their treatment, education, and research programs.

The Arthritis Foundation has headquarters in Atlanta and 72 chapters nationwide. The Arthritis Society has national headquarters in Toronto and 10 divisions spanning Canada. These are the only agencies devoted to searching for the underlying causes and subsequent cures for arthritis while promoting the best possible care for arthritis sufferers. In addition they offer information, materials, and group programs.

Arthritis Foundation
National Office
P.O. Box 19000
Atlanta, GA 30309

Arthritis Society
250 Bloor St., East
Suite 401
Toronto, Ontario
Canada M4W 3P2

For regional offices, look in your telephone book under Arthritis Foundation or Arthritis Society.

ABOUT THE AUTHOR

Gwen Ellert was born and raised in Vancouver, Canada. She obtained her bachelor of science degree in nursing from the University of British Columbia in 1974. In 1973 Gwen was diagnosed as having rheumatoid arthritis. As a result of this disease she had a total knee and ankle replacement in the late 1970s and had to give up tennis, snow skiing, water skiing, and playing the guitar.

Since the time of her diagnosis, Gwen has been involved in a multidisciplinary treatment program. Recovery has been slow but steady and Gwen believes that this is the result of the correct combination of medication, rest, and exercise.

Gwen's determination, enthusiasm for life, and love of people have enabled her to pursue many goals: design and teach night-school classes in medical terminology, write this book, and maintain a demanding career. *The Arthritis Exercise Book* reflects Gwen's work and interest in public health education.

ABOUT THE CONSULTANT

Gillian Parker is a physiotherapist specializing in arthritis since 1972. After heading the Arthritis Service at G. F. Strong Rehabilitation Centre in Vancouver, Canada, for nine years, she joined the B.C. Arthritis Society, working as the education physiotherapist from 1982 to 1985. She developed and provided education programs for patients, peers, and the general public.

Born in England, Ms. Parker was raised in South Africa and graduated as a physiotherapist in 1964 from the University of Cape Town. Ms. Parker immigrated to Canada in 1966. She retired from her position with the Arthritis Society in 1985 to raise a family and presently maintains a keen interest and involvement in her professional specialty.

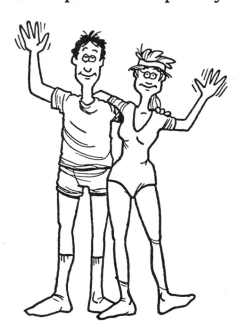